The Holy Bible of Superfoods

DEDICATION

This book is dedicated to my beautiful children Seven and Serenity, and my loving wife Danielle whom in her dual multi-talented nature for bringing my work to life. I also would like to dedicate this book to my grandfather Walter Hamm (my first Hero) and my Dearest Aunt, Geraldine Blanks.

TABLE OF CONTENTS

ACKNOWLEDGMENTS

First and foremost, I would like to acknowledge and thank each and every client, co-worker, advisor, and those whom I have personally helped along their journeys throughout the years healing various ailments.

God Created a Seed

And in this Seed

Every kind of Plant Food will grow

The Father of Jesus said, "Come forwardth fruits, nuts, veggies, beans, and grains".

In man, the Father of Jesus made man and woman to eat to live "One Bite at a Time".

Welcome to the Holy

BIBLE of

SUPERFOODS

The ULTIMATE DRIVING MACHINE is your body and it is designed to transport your mind through space and time. The only way to do that in a healthy way is to eat Superfoods consistently.

IN THE BIBLE…

Genesis 1:29 – 30

Then God said, "I give you every seed – bearing plant on the face of the whole earth and every tree that has a fruit with seeds in it. They will be yours for food and to all the beasts of the earth, and all the birds of the air, and all the creatures that move on the ground – everything that has the breath of life. In it, I give every green plant for food and it was so".

LOVE, NOT EAT our ANIMALS, for after we eat them. They start to eat your health away, ESPECIALLY when you are eating meat on a daily basis.

What is a Superfood? Superfoods are foods loaded with mega minerals and nutrients, proteins, and antioxidants. Superfoods are God's technology known for healing and enhancing your mood, health, and energy.

The Heavenly Father created Superfoods for Supernatural people. Once your taste buds get touched by SUPERFOODS, you will notice how good you will feel and how life is extended just by eating healthier!

WELCOME TO THE GARDEN OF SUPERFOODS...

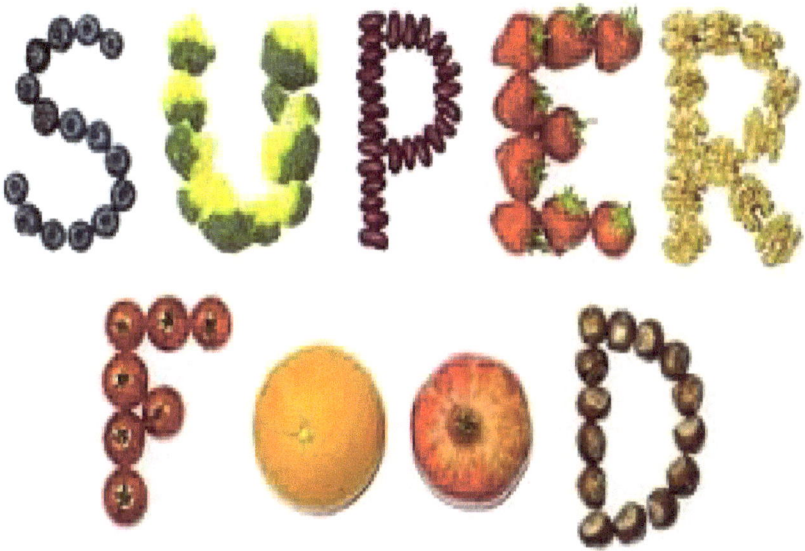

"FRUITS"

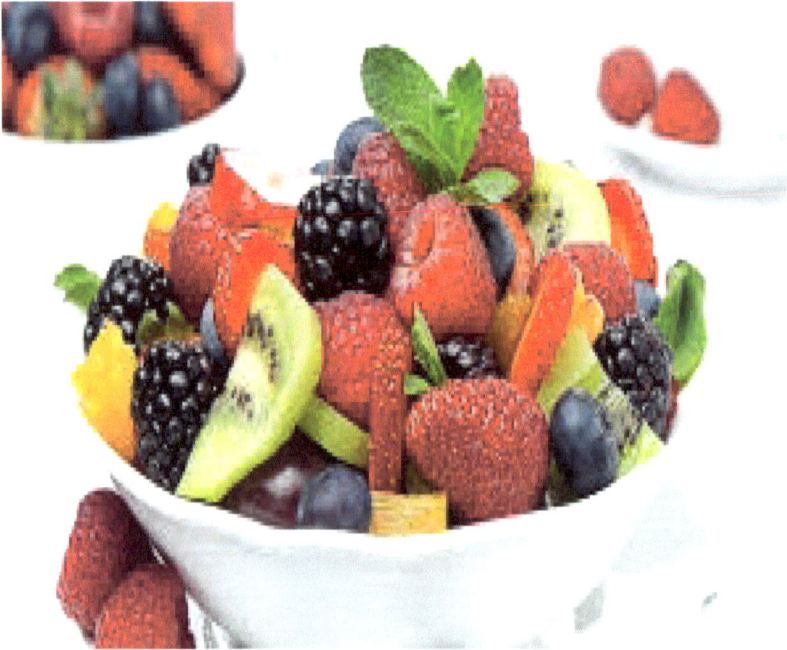

ACAI BERRIES

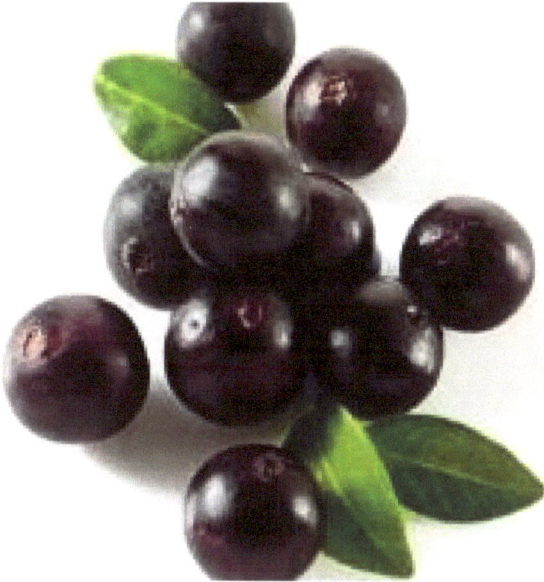

ACAI BERRIES are one of the most potent fruits on the planet! It is loaded with antioxidants, lowers your cholesterol, in addition to having anti-cancer healing properties. They improve your sexual libido. Acai berries also aides in improving your cognitive skills. This is a very powerful food. The Acai Berry is hard to obtain in the United States of America. However, they can be found in Central and South America. This fruit is medicinal. These berries grow in huge clusters near the tops of palm trees in the Amazon rain forests. They also are high in fiber and heart-healthy fats.

APPLES

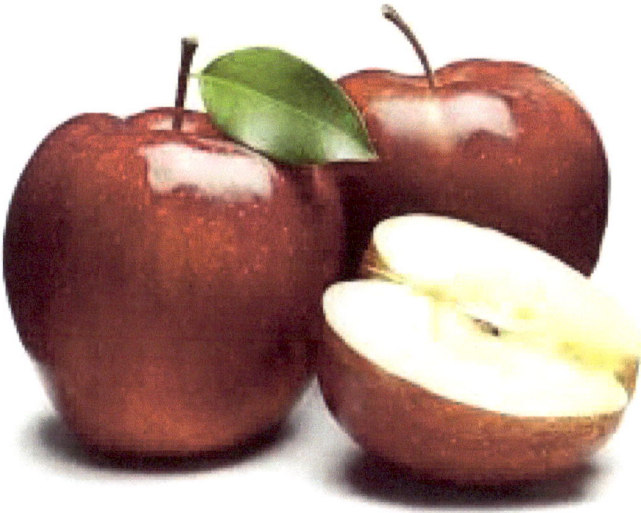

APPLES are one of the most popular fruits on the planet. They're an exceptionally healthy fruit. It's packed with vitamins C&K, potassium and fiber. Apples promote weight loss. They are also good for your heart as it aides in lowering your cholesterol. They have also been linked to lowering the risk of diabetes. Apples ripen six to 10 times faster at room temperature than if they are refrigerated. They float in water because they are 25% air.

AVOCADO

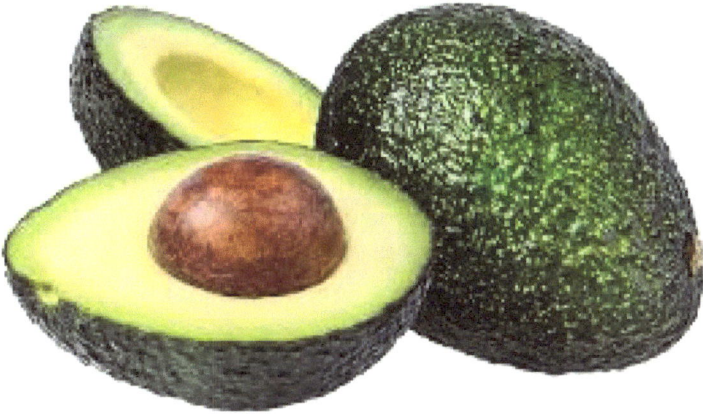

AVOCADOS are a very powerful superfood known for lowering your cholesterol. They are loaded with fiber and have more potassium then bananas. They are rich in antioxidants that can protect your eyes. Avocado increases the libido. They are loaded with fiber. It is an anti-cancer food, so it boosts the immune system. Avocados are loaded with heart healthy monounsaturated fatty acids. I love to eat it with toast in the morning or blended in with my smoothie ingredients.

BLACKBERRIES

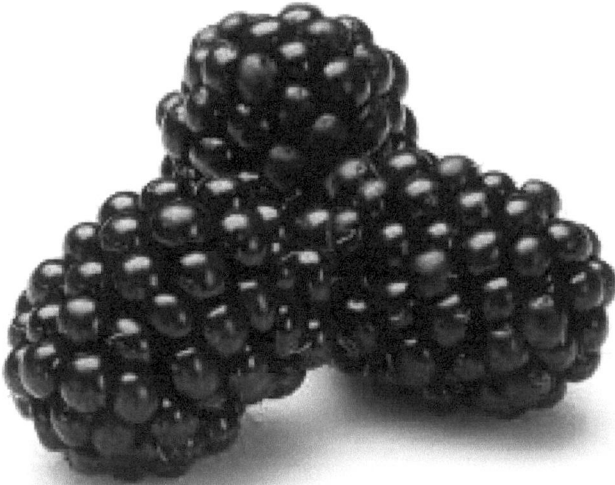

BLACKBERRIES are an antioxidant which are excellent for immune and oral health because they are loaded with vitamins C and K. They are also a great source of fiber. Blackberries can help with a woman's menstruation, stabilizing her hormones. Instead of taking supplements, eat a handful of blackberries. Like all superfoods, blackberries are an anti-inflammatory food. They also assist with improving brain functioning. Blackberries also support oral health.

CHERRIES

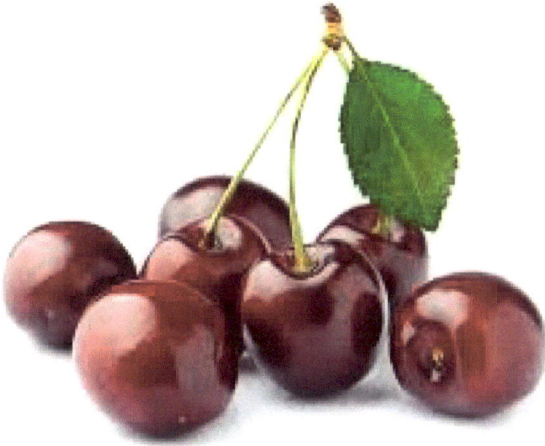

CHERRIES like all superfoods, are loaded with antioxidants. They also have anti-inflammatory properties. Cherries are a good source of fiber, vitamin A and minerals including potassium, calcium, and folic acid. They help to relax you to sleep better at night. They also bring relief to arthritis and gout. They also lower the risk of a heart attack and strokes.

CUCUMBER

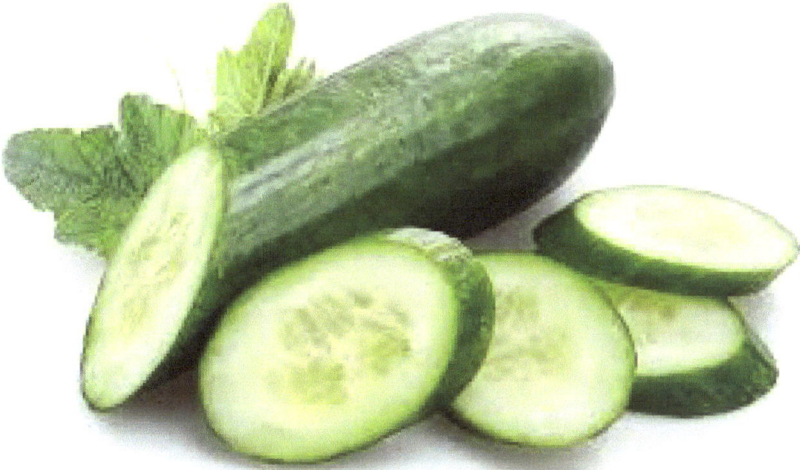

CUCUMBERS are one of my favorite fruits. They are loaded with vitamins B1, B2, B3, B5, & B6. They also contain vitamin c, iron, calcium, magnesium, phosphorus, and potassium. Cucumbers are known to cure bad breath. They have been linked to reducing the risk of developing breast, ovarian, colon, and prostate cancers. Pureed or sliced cucumbers give an almost instant relief to sunburnt skin. Just place some against the affected area.

GRAPEFRUIT

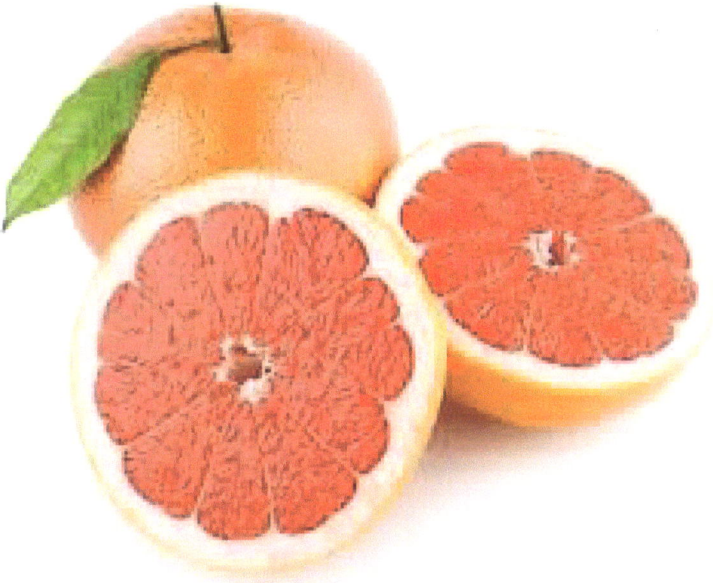

GRAPEFRUITS are very low in calories, yet high in nutrients. It's high in powerful antioxidants. They are very beneficial to your immune system. Grapefruits also promote appetite control and weight loss. Eating grapefruits regularly may have the potential to prevent insulin resistance, which can lead to diabetes. They also improve heart health reducing the risk factors for heart disease, such as high blood pressure and cholesterol.

Grapefruits may reduce the risk of kidney stones. Grapefruits contains a lot of water and is, therefore, very hydrating. In fact, water makes up most of the fruit's weight.

GRAPES *with* SEEDS

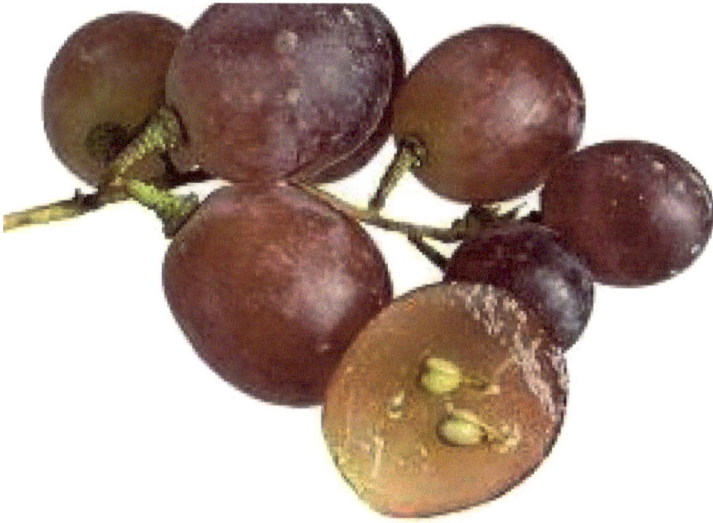

GRAPES with seeds of all colors are a natural source of antioxidants and other polyphenols that offer a variety of additional health benefits. Grapes are an excellent source of vitamins C&K. Like all fruits, grapes have no cholesterol. They have anti-cancer fighting properties. Grapes boosts your immunity, regulates the blood pressure and are good for the eyes. Due to its high potassium content and low quantum of sodium grapes help maintain the electrolyte balance of the body and flush out excess water and toxins. The abundant antioxidants present in grapes help prevent atherosclerosis or hardening of the arteries. They are also great for pain relief and inflammation.

KIWI

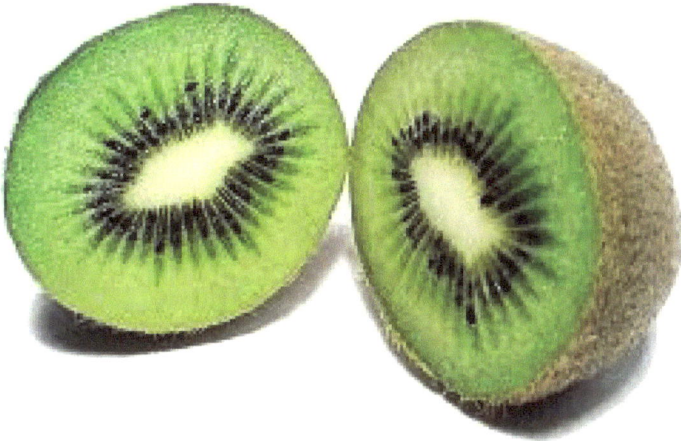

KIWIS are a great aide to help treat asthma. They are also an aide in digestion. Kiwi's are packed with antioxidants and vitamin C. They boost the immune system and reduces the risk of other health conditions. Not only can kiwi fruits aide in managing blood pressure, they reduce blood clotting as well.

They protect against vision loss. Since oxidative DNA damage is strongly linked to colon cancer, regular kiwi consumption could lower the risk of colon cancer.

LIME

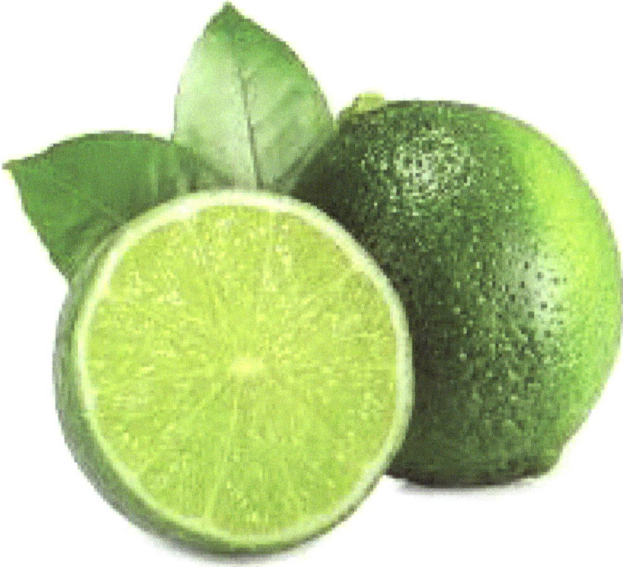

LIMES are a great source of antioxidants. They are high in vitamin C, a nutrient that helps boost your immune system. They promote healthy skin as well. Limes aide in reducing the risk of heart disease. They prevent kidney stones and increase iron absorption. They have also been known to lower the risk of certain cancers.

LEMON

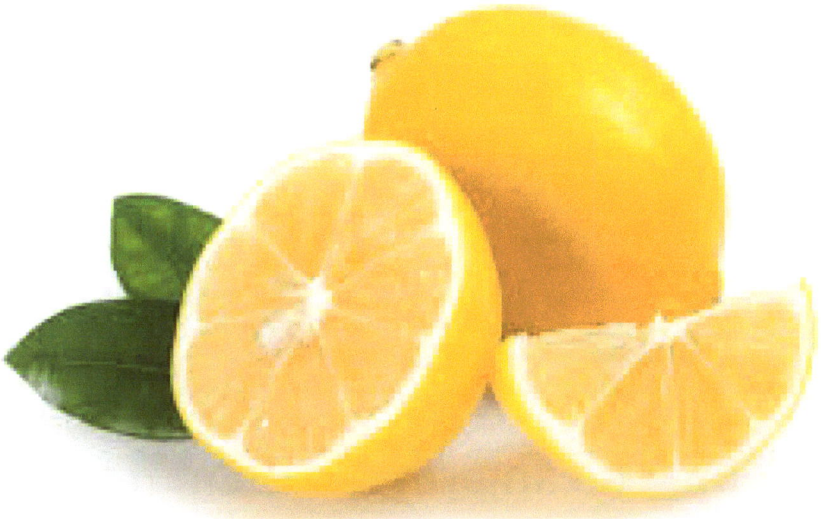

LEMONS are a very popular and delicious fruit. They are an antioxidant, so they will boost the immune system. They are also known for reducing the risk of cancer while preventing kidney stones. Lemons are great for combatting the common cold as they are rich in vitamin C. The high acidity in lemons make them a great cleaning aide. Each lemon contains approximately 15 calories. An average lemon holds three tablespoons of lemon juice. One trick that I learned is if you sprinkle the juice of a lemon on to other fruits, it can prevent them from turning brown.

MANGO

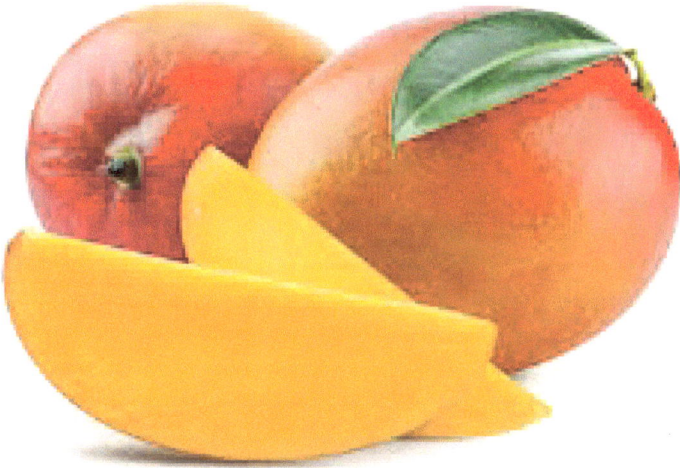

MANGOS like all other superfoods are high in antioxidants which aides in eye health. They are packed with vitamins A, B, C, and K. Mangos also have approximately 1 gram of protein. They are anti-cancer food that increases bone health, aide in fighting diabetes and heart disease. In addition, mangos are great for hair growth and clears your skin from deep inside the body. It treats pores and gives a glow to your skin. Mangos help in controlling high cholesterol levels. My son Seven love's them!

POMEGRANATE

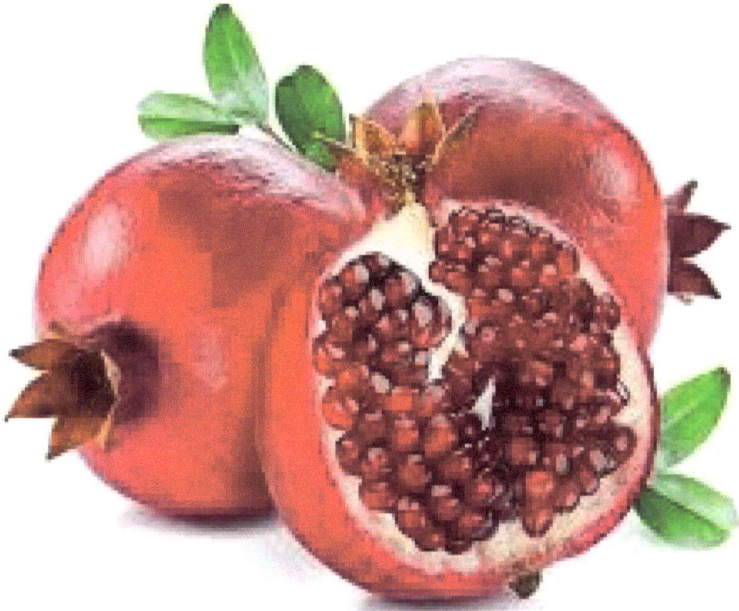

POMERGRANATES are an antioxidant that has anti-inflammatory properties. This superfood provides the ultimate driving machine which is the BODY with healing properties.

Pomegranate seeds get their vibrant hue from polyphenols. These chemicals are powerful antioxidants. Pomegranates provide vitamin C, aid to prevent cancer as well as shield against Alzheimer's Disease, and Arthritis. Additionally, it boosts the immune system, remove free radicals, protect cells from damage, and aids against Heart Disease.

Have one and share it with your family!

PRUNES

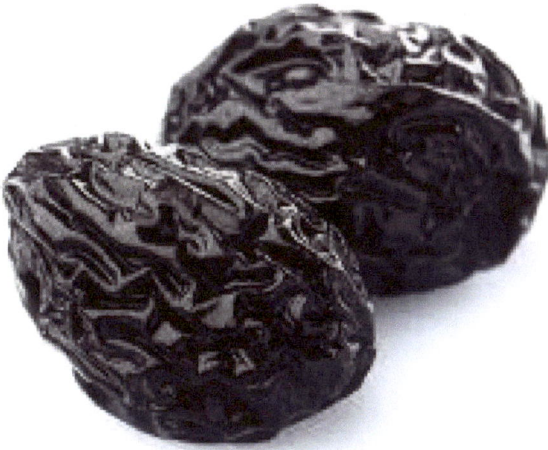

PRUNES are very rich in antioxidants and great for digestive health. They help to reduce cholesterol levels, lower your blood sugar levels and a great source of iron and vitamins K, A, B2, and B3. Prunes also aid in building bones and muscles. Known for being high in fiber, it is highly encouraged that "meat eaters" annually cleanse out your colon with this drink or eating the actual fruit to reduce the risk of colon malfunction. Prunes have several characteristics that may reduce the risk of many chronic diseases, such as osteoporosis, cancer, heart disease and diabetes.

RASPBERRIES

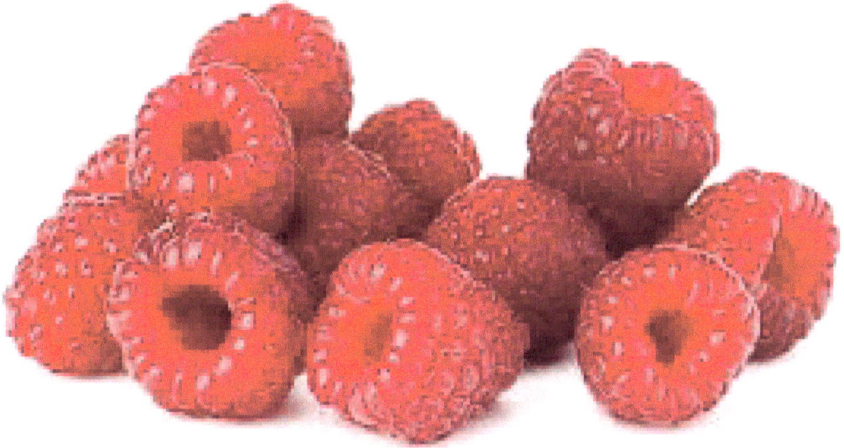

RASPBERRIES are low in calories and packed with nutrients. They also have cancer-fighting properties. They aide in weight loss and combat aging by fighting free radicals in your body. Raspberries have anti-inflammatory properties which aide in reducing symptoms of arthritis. They protect against diabetes.

STRAWBERRIES

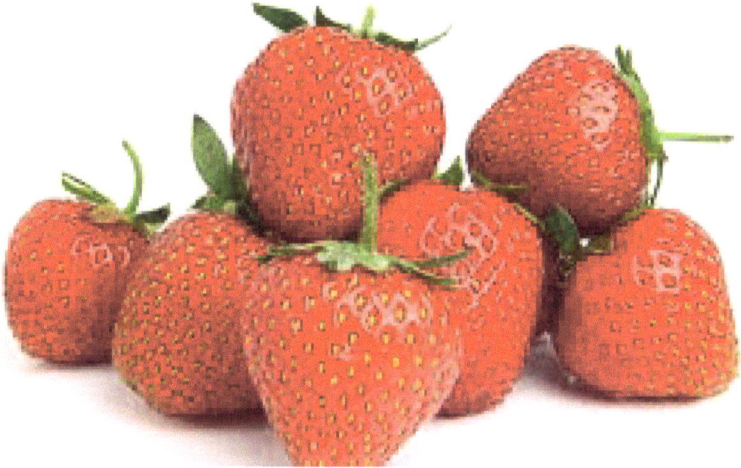

STRAWBERRIES are high in antioxidants. They are excellent for improving heart health and promoting a happy mood. Strawberries aide in preventing strokes and cancer as well. They help to lower your blood pressure in addition to being an anti-inflammatory food. Strawberries are high in water content and fiber that hydrates the body and helps to maintain regular bowel movements. They are a helpful fruit choice for people living with diabetes.

TOMATOES

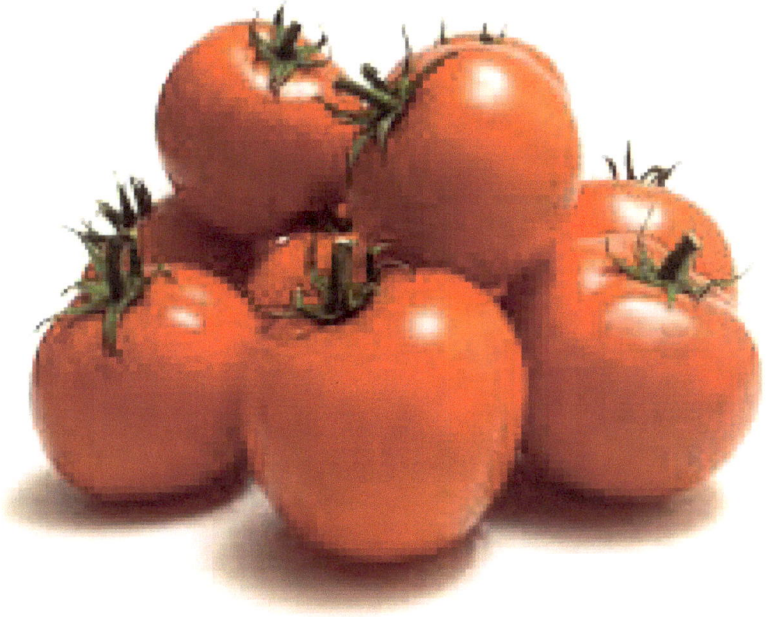

TOMATOES are a great source of vitamins C & K, potassium, and folate, amongst other powerful antioxidants. They are great for heart health. Tomatoes aide in preventing cancer and are beneficial for skin health. They help to lower your blood pressure. Tomatoes also aide in preventing diabetes, and constipation. They have been known to protect they eyes against light-induced damage and are great for the skin.

Although many people think that tomatoes are a vegetable as they are very popular in salads, they are definitely a fruit, as they contain seeds!

WATERMELON with SEEDS

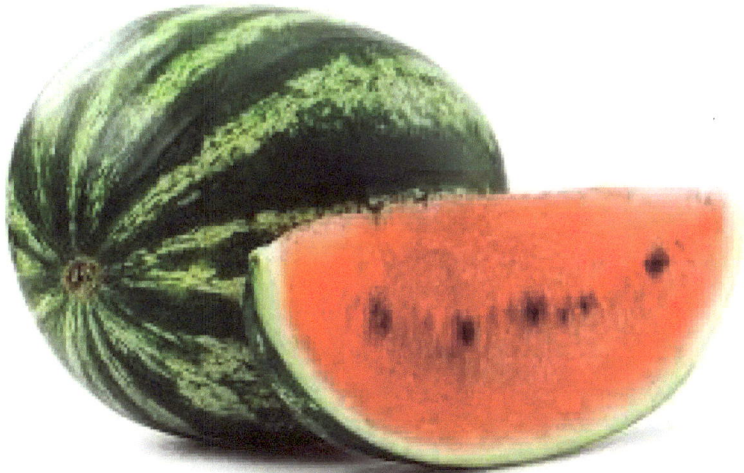

WATERMELONS are a stress reliever. It contains compounds that may help to prevent cancer. It hydrates the body. It also aide muscle soreness while boosting your immune system. Watermelons are packed with vitamins A, C, and B. It is good for the skin and hair. This superfood also battles inflammation and promotes heart health. It helps to lower oxidative stress. Watermelon with seeds are one of my all-time favorite holy foods. It also boosts your libido and helps to improve your digestive system.

"NUTS"

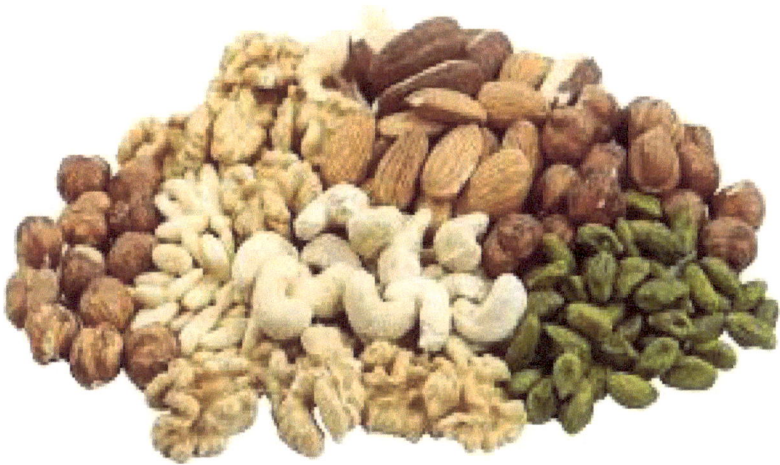

ALMONDS

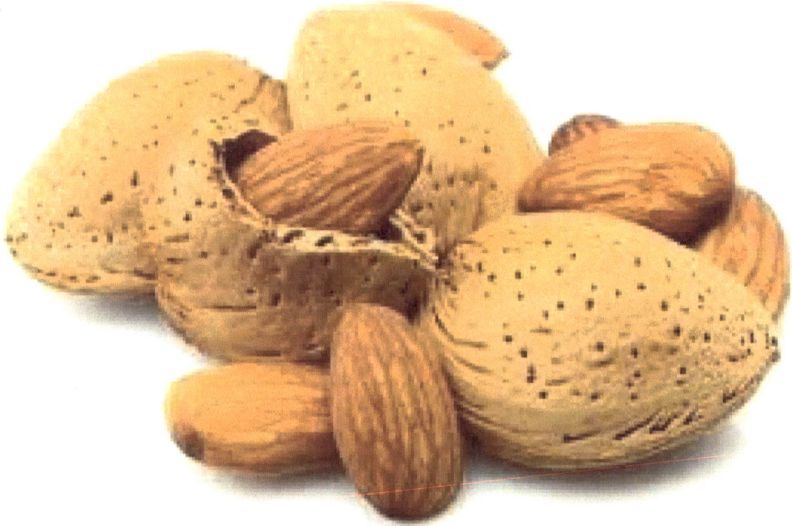

ALMONDS are among the world's most popular tree nuts. They are highly nutritious and rich in healthy fats, antioxidants, vitamins and minerals. The powerful antioxidants in almonds are largely concentrated in brown layer of the skin. Almonds can assist with blood sugar and pressure levels. This makes them the perfect choice for people with diabetes. Almonds can lower your cholesterol levels too. Eating almonds reduce hunger while lowering your overall calorie intake. Almonds promote weight loss. They taste great covered in dark chocolate too!

BRAZIL NUTS

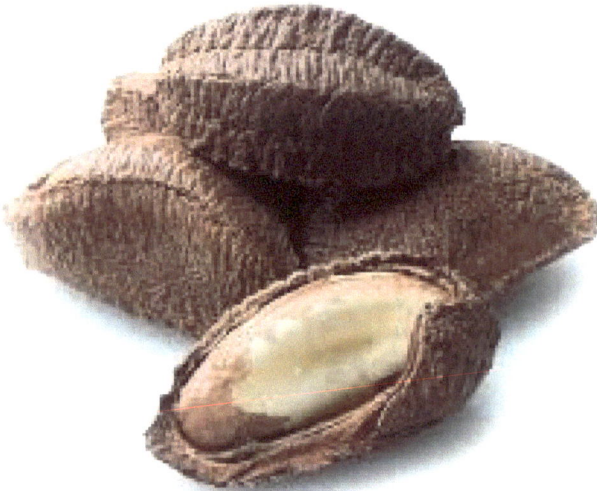

BRAZIL NUTS are great for your heart. The calcium, magnesium, and potassium in brazil nuts can help to regulate blood pressure. They also aide in lowering cholesterol levels. Brazil nuts are a good source of an antioxidant called selenium which help to keep disease at bay and are specifically linked to lowering the risk of heart disease. They're a good source of copper, which helps to build tissue and generate energy in the cells. These nuts support the nervous system. You don't have to eat a lot of them to make a big impact on you daily nutrient requirements. Brazil nuts are considered a "complete" protein as it is combined with all nine amino acids.

WALNUTS

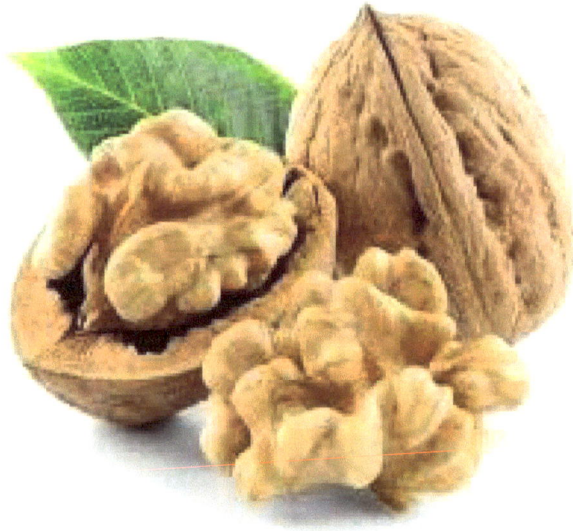

WALNUTS have the highest level of antioxidants compared to most common nuts. They help to lower the blood pressure, aid in Type 2 Diabetes. Walnuts can also decrease inflammation. They are known for promoting a healthy stomach. Also, walnuts are great for improved bone health. They help to increase a better mood in women and children while supporting male reproductive health. Walnuts have approximately 15% protein. They are a super plant source of Omega-3s. Walnuts may also reduce the risk of some cancers. They also promote weight control. Walnuts also support good brain function and improve blood fats. I love to eat them raw and unsalted.

"VEGGIES"

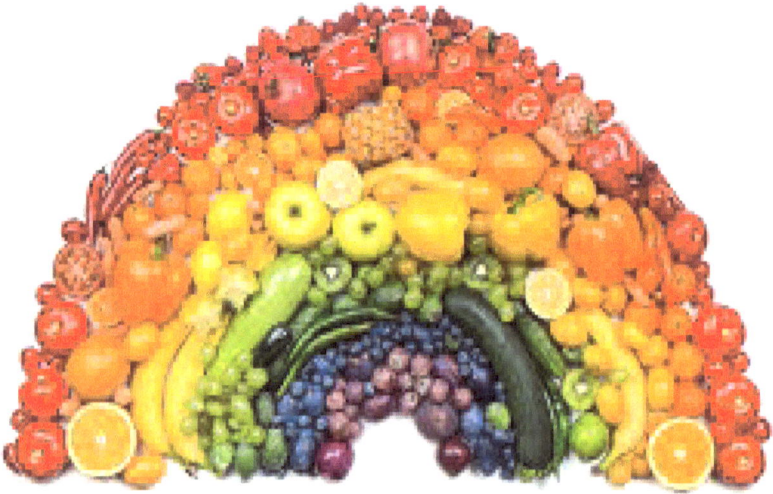

ASPARAGUS

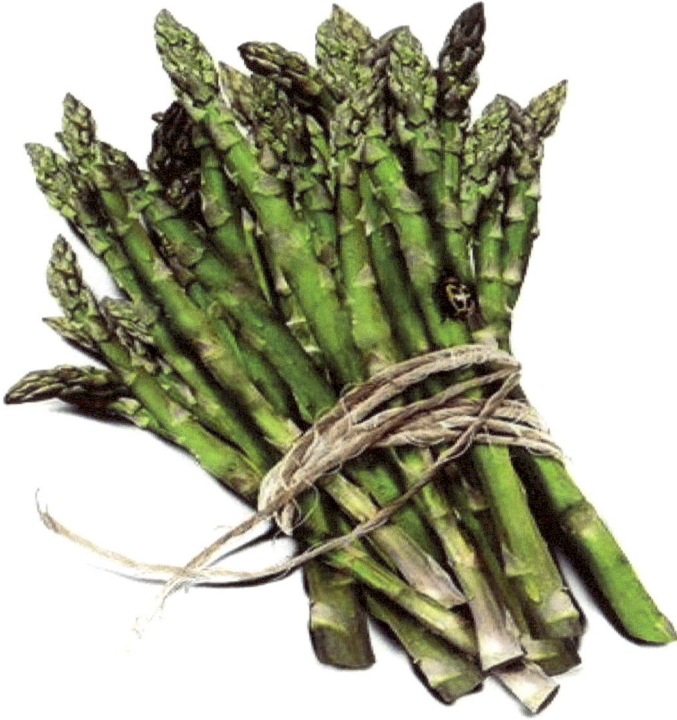

ASPARAGUS is a low-calorie vegetable that is an excellent source of essential vitamins and minerals, especially folate and vitamins A, C, and K. In addition, asparagus is high in folate, a nutrient that is vital for a healthy pregnancy and many important processes in the body, including cell growth and DNA formation. Asparagus aides in improving digestive health. They also assist in lowering blood pressure levels. This powerful antioxidant can help you to lose weight.

BOK CHOY

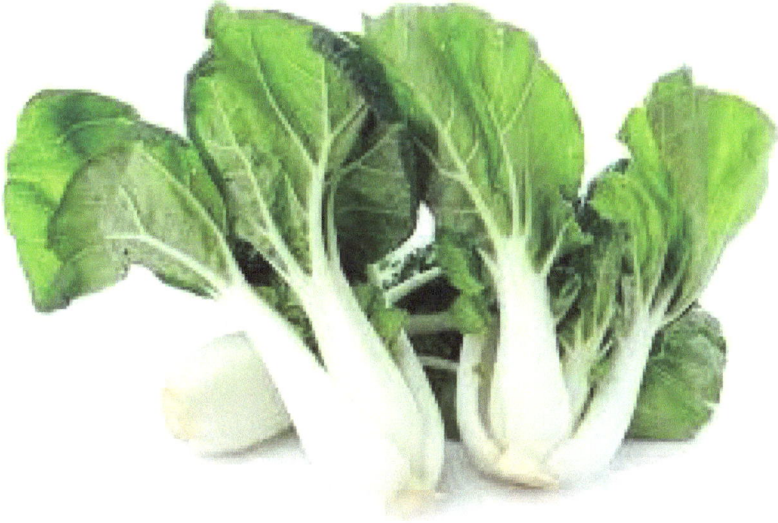

BOK CHOY has anti-cancer properties. This vegetable is packed with vitamins C & E and beta-carotene. These nutrients have powerful antioxidant properties that help protect cells against damage by free radicals. Bok Choy aides in bone health. It also can decrease blood pressure. They are great for heart health and helps to reduce inflammation. Boy Choy is great for the skin's support system. It helps to maintain blood sugar levels. The selenium found in Bok Choy has been found to improve immune response to infection by stimulating the production of T-cells that identify and kill invading bacteria and viruses.

BRUSSEL SPROUTS

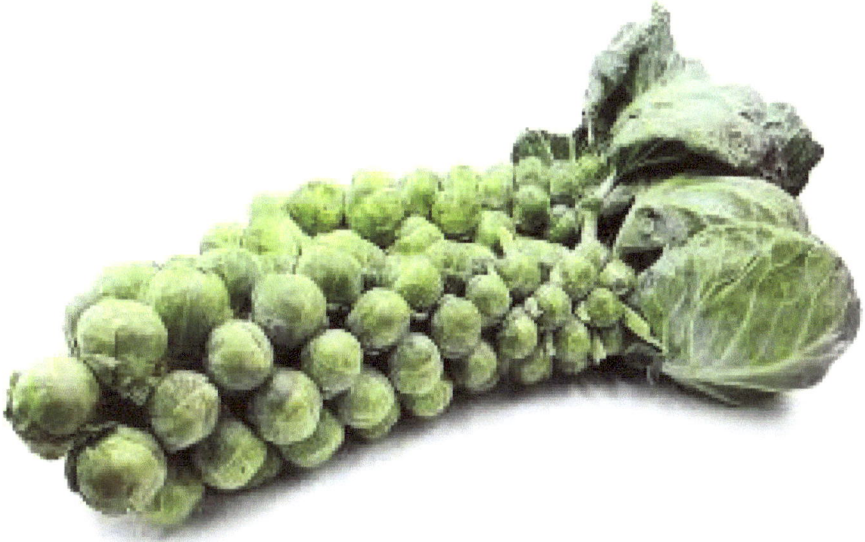

BRUSSEL SPROUTS are high in nutrients like vitamins K, C, and A. They are high in fiber and protects against cancer. They help to maintain healthy blood sugar levels. Brussel Sprouts are also a great source of Omega 3s fatty acids while helping to reduce the risk of inflammation. They even contain protein. They taste great cooked or raw.

CABBAGE

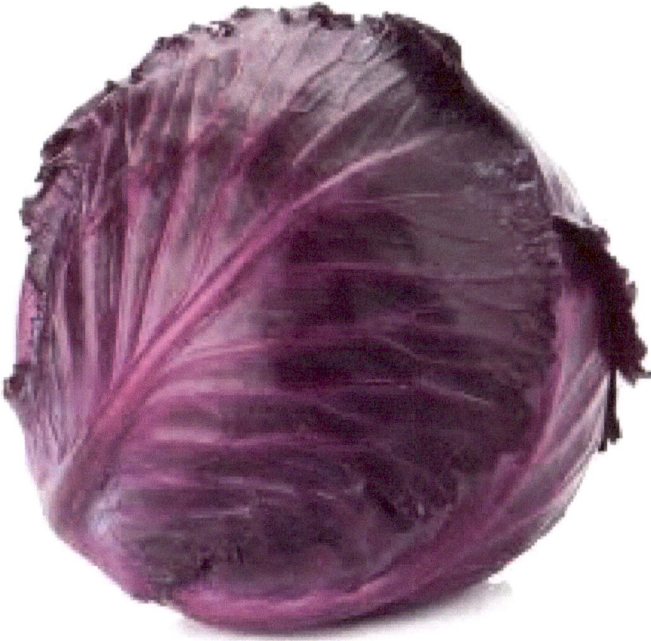

CABBAGE is packed with nutrients. It is rich in vitamins B6, C, K, and folate, both of which are essential for many important processes in the body, including energy metabolism and the normal functioning of the nervous system. It helps keep inflammation in check. Cabbage also aides in improving digestion. This is a heart healthy vegetable that assists in lowering blood pressure and cholesterol levels. Eating cabbage helps lower the risk of certain diseases, improve digestion and combats inflammation.

GARLIC

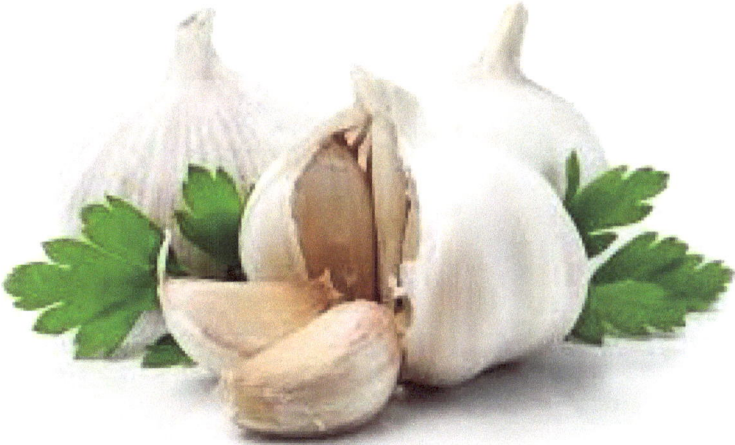

GARLIC contains compounds with potent medicinal properties. It is a very powerful superfood packed with manganese, vitamins B6 and C. Garlic reduces the risk of heart disease. Also, it's known for lowering blood pressure and cholesterol. Garlic can be used to combat sickness, including the common cold. It contains antioxidants that may help prevent Alzheimer's Disease and Dementia. It aides in life longevity and improves bone health.

GREEN BEANS

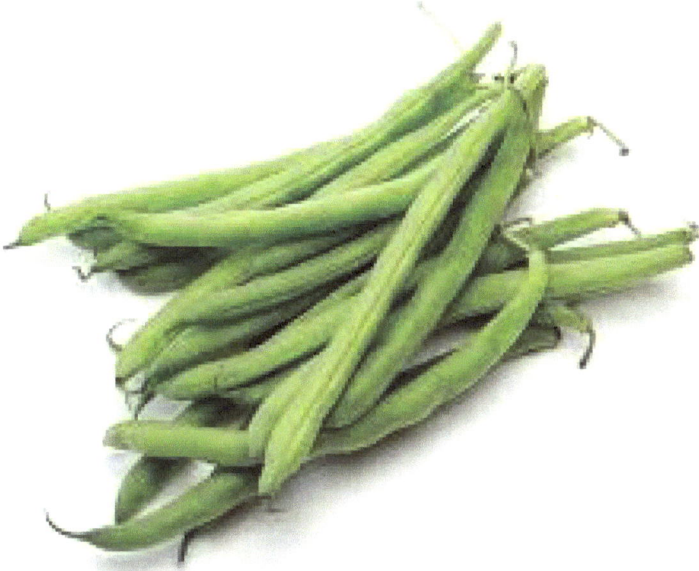

GREEN BEANS also called "snap beans" or "string beans" help you maintain a healthy weight. They contain no cholesterol. Green beans are heart healthy by lowering blood pressure and reducing inflammation. Green beans contain protein which is essential to a healthy immune system. One cup of raw green beans has almost 2 grams of protein. Green beans are a good source of vitamins A, B, C, E, & K, folate, and minerals including manganese. This essential mineral supports your metabolism and has antioxidant abilities.

KALE

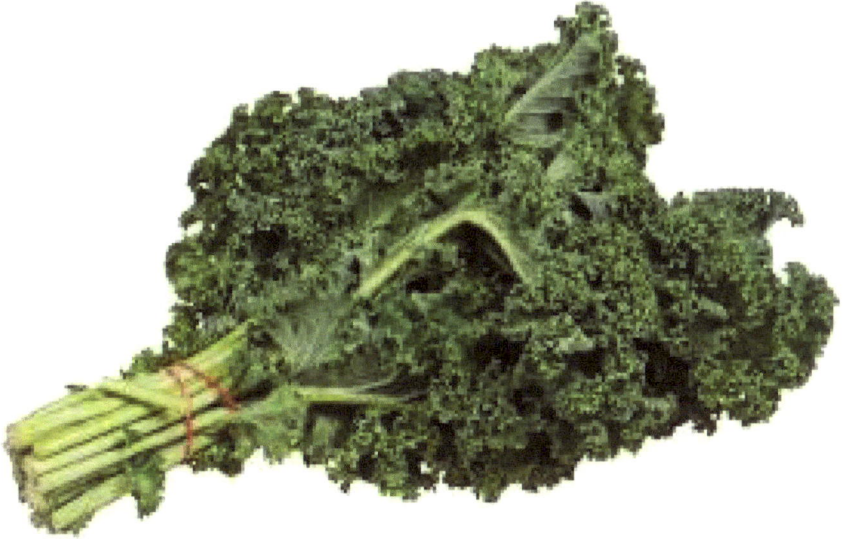

KALE is among the most nutrient-dense vegetables on the planet. Kale, like other leafy greens, is very high in antioxidants. It is an excellent source of vitamins C & K that serves many vital functions in the body's cells. Kale can help lower cholesterol levels, which reduces the risk of heart disease.

Kale can boost your well being by renewing your skin cells and tissues. There are numerous cancer-fighting substances in Kale. It aides in eye protection. Kale has several properties that make it a weight loss friendly vegetable.

"Lightly sprinkled in olive oil and Himalayan salt placed into the oven for about 7 minutes makes great Kale chips."

RED ONION

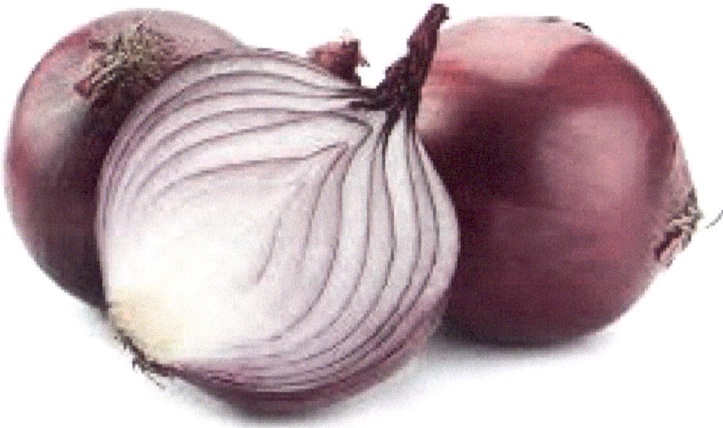

RED ONIONS have many health benefits like reducing the risk of cancer, obesity, heart disease and arthritis. In addition, red onions kill bacteria, boosts the immune system, and are loaded with antioxidants, minerals, and vitamins B and C. Red onions are a very good source of biotin. They are also a great source of manganese. I eat them both raw and cooked.

RED SKINNED POTATOES

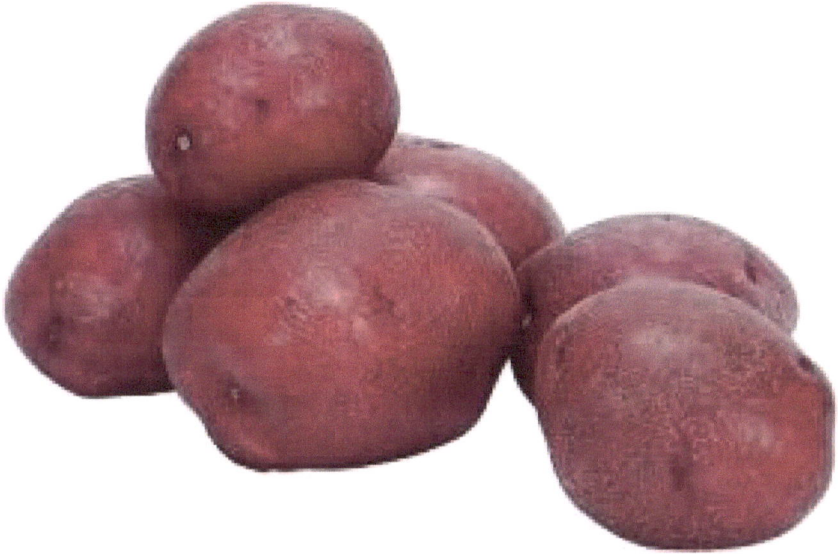

RED SKINNED POTATOES are my families favorite. They are a great source of vitamins B6 & C, iron and helps to repair body tissue and providing antioxidants. Red skinned potatoes have more potassium than a banana. They are also packed with fiber. Much of the nutritional value of a potato is found in its skin.

Red skinned potatoes also aide in lowering stress levels. They increase your energy. They are naturally fat free. Red skinned potatoes also help to maintain a healthy blood pressure.

SEAWEED

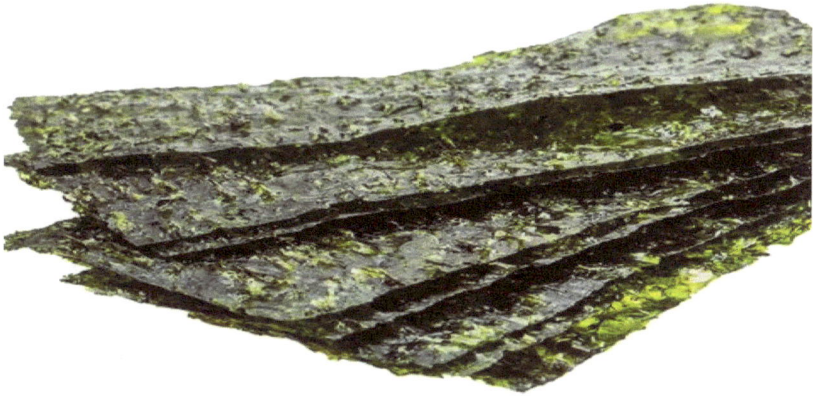

SEAWEED contains Iodine and Tyrosine, which supports thyroid function. It is a great source of vitamins and minerals such as vitamin K, B vitamins, zinc and iron with antioxidants that help protect your cells from damage. Seaweed is also packed with omega-3 fats.

Seaweed is an excellent source of fiber, which is known to promote gut health. The fiber in seaweed may slow stomach emptying, too. This helps you feel fuller for longer and delays hunger pangs. It reduces the risk of heart disease and improves blood sugar levels.

SUGAR SNAP PEAS

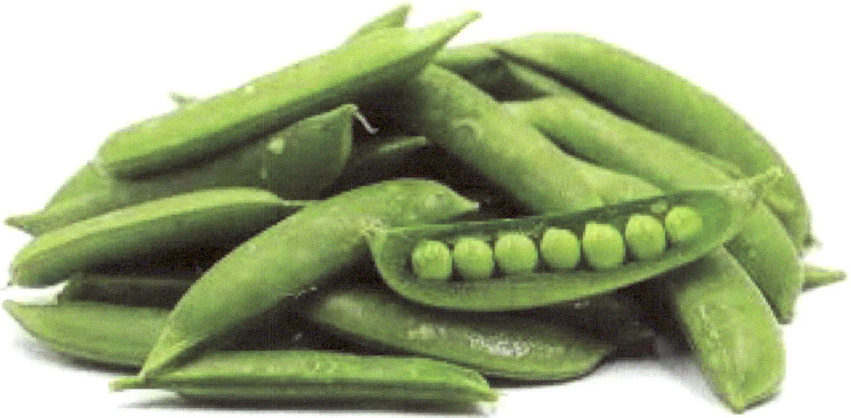

SUGAR SNAP PEAS, like other edible pea pods, deliver many of the key nutrients needed for good health. They improve digestive and heart function while aiding in the metabolism of fats and blood sugars. Snap peas also help you meet some of your vitamin and mineral needs, including vitamin C, folate and potassium. It is very rich in iron too. It is also an antioxidant that protects your cells from free radicals. This little treat is naturally sweet and tasty.

SPINACH

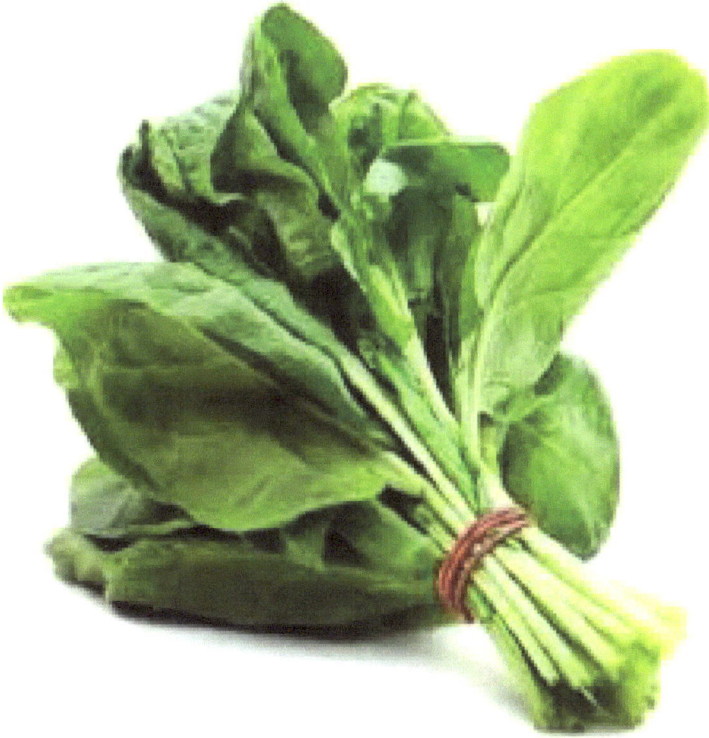

SPINACH is one of the most popular green, leafy vegetables in the world as it is a rich source of vitamins and minerals. The nitrates in spinach can potentially improve athletic performance, reduce cholesterol levels, and lessen the risk of heart disease. Nitrates may also help lower blood sugar levels. Spinach reduces the risk of cancer. One cup of raw spinach contains approximately 1 gram of protein. Besides its high protein content, spinach contains plant compounds that can increase antioxidant defense and reduce inflammation. Eating spinach may benefit eye health and reduce oxidative stress levels. Spinach is high in vitamin K1, which serves several functions in your body but is best known for its role in blood clotting.

SWEET POTATOES

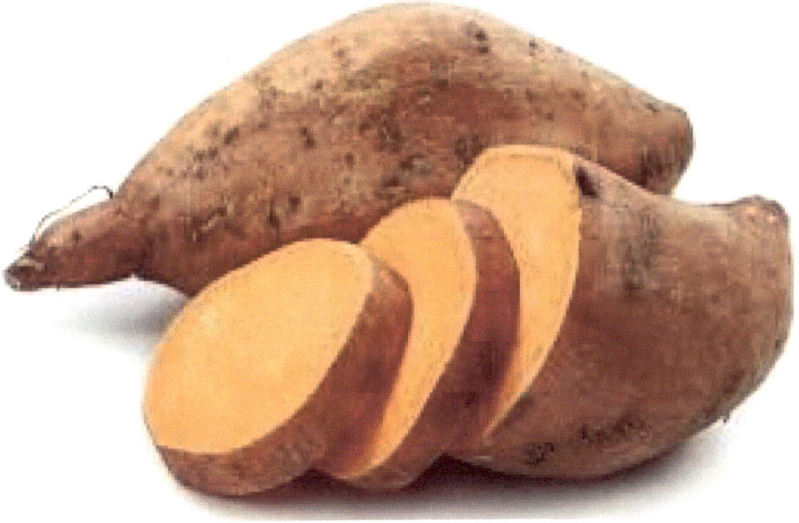

SWEET POTATOES pack a powerful nutritional punch! In one medium spud, there is over 400 percent of your daily vitamin A requirement. Sweet potatoes also contain high amounts of fiber and potassium. They promote gut health. Sweet potatoes have cancer-fighting properties. They also support healthy vision and enhance brain function. Sweet potatoes are rich in beta-carotene, a plant-based compound that is converted to vitamin a in your body which aides in supporting your immune system.

SWISS CHARD

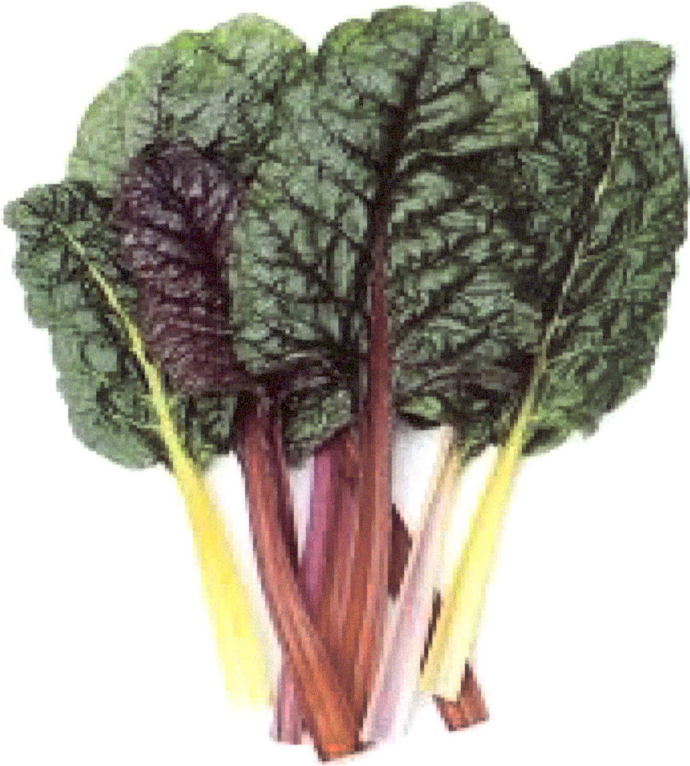

SWISS CHARD is a superfood that's loaded with both proteins and disease fighting antioxidants. It is one of the healthiest leafy green vegetables. It is a great source of vitamins K, A, and C. In addition to being an awesome source of magnesium, Swiss Chard is high in potassium, iron, and fiber. It may decrease insulin resistance and lower your blood sugar. Swiss Chard promotes weight loss. It can be prepared in many different ways. *"I love eating it raw in a super salad."*

"BEANS"

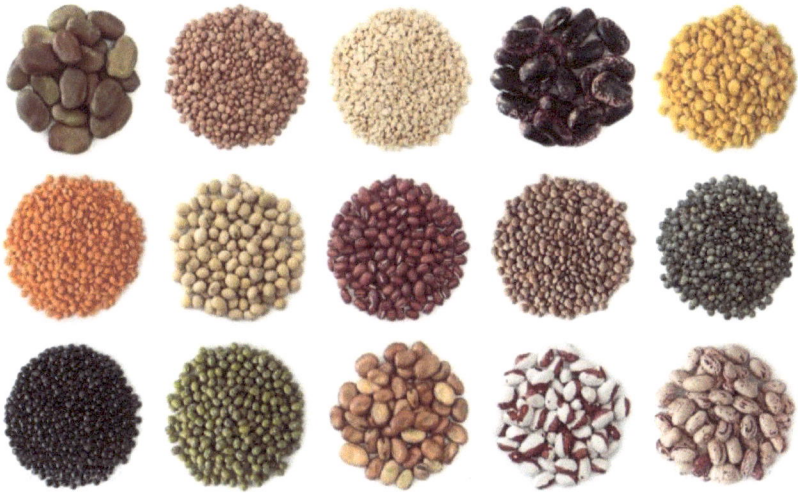

BLACK BEANS

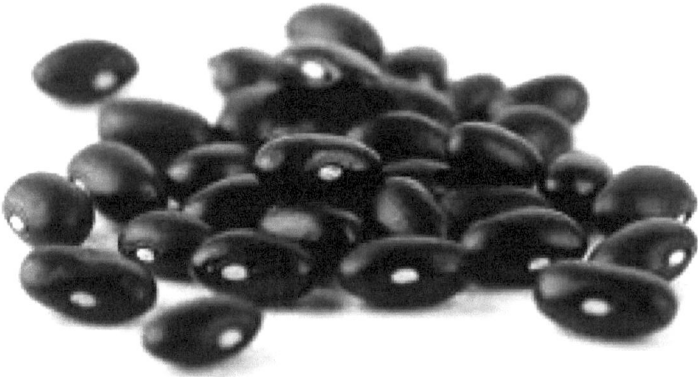

BLACK BEANS are high in protein and fiber properties. They renew skin cells and tissues, increase libido in men and promote healthy hair growth. They are also known to reduce the chances of cancer and weight loss. Black beans aide in maintaining healthy bones. They also assist in lowering your blood pressure and managing diabetes. Because of the fiber content, black beans help to prevent constipation and promote regularity for a healthy digestive tract.

EDAMAME

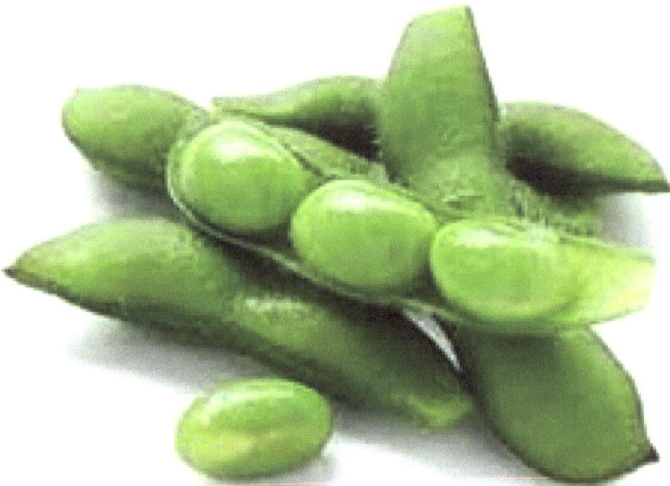

EDAMAME is high in protein. They aides in lowering cholesterol levels. These beans are great for people with diabetes. They are packed with vitamins and minerals. Edamame aides in reducing the risk of breast cancer. They also reduce menopausal symptoms and the risk of prostate cancer. They aide in reducing bone loss as well. They are the cornerstone of many vegan and vegetarian diets.

LENTIL BEANS

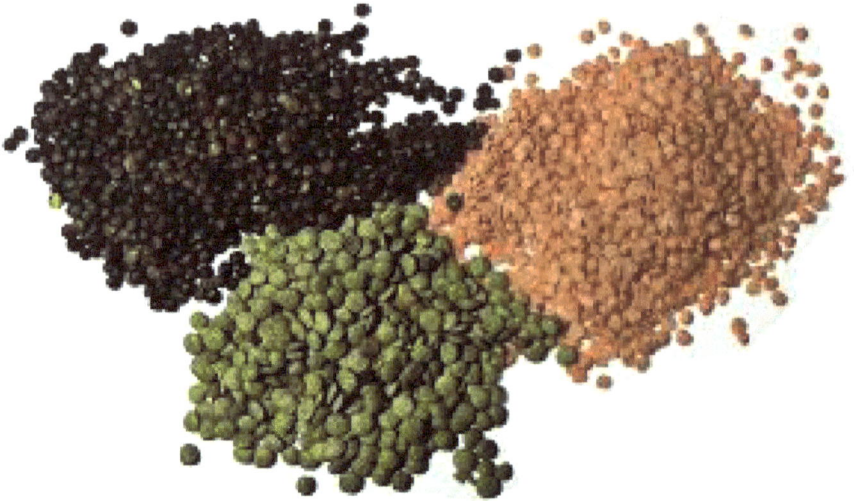

LENTIL BEANS come in various colors and are minerally rich with fiber, vitamin B, magnesium, zinc, and potassium. They are great for meat substituting as they are made up of over 25% protein. Lentil Beans cook in under 35 minutes and inherit healthy benefits like lowering your blood pressure and cholesterol. Eating lentils is associated with an overall lower risk of heart disease. In addition to increasing a man's libido.

RED KIDNEY BEANS

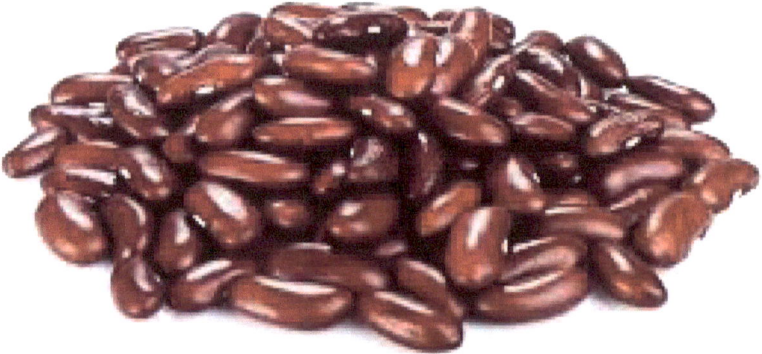

RED KIDNEY BEANS are great for reducing fatty liver. They improve your heart and brain function. Being both a protein and antioxidant, red beans lower your cholesterol and fight fatigue. Red Kidney Beans are rich in vitamin K1 which is very important for blood coagulation. They also promote weight loss and improve your blood sugar levels. It also aides in preventing colon cancer.

"GRAINS"

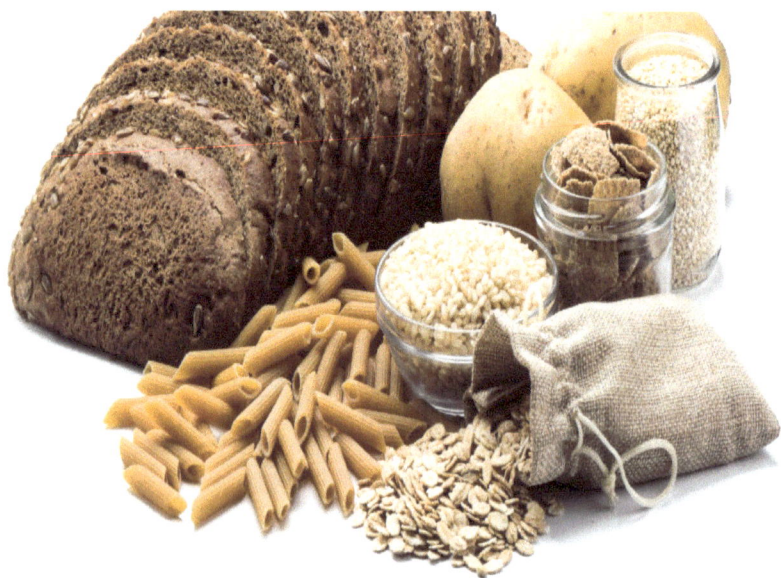

OATS

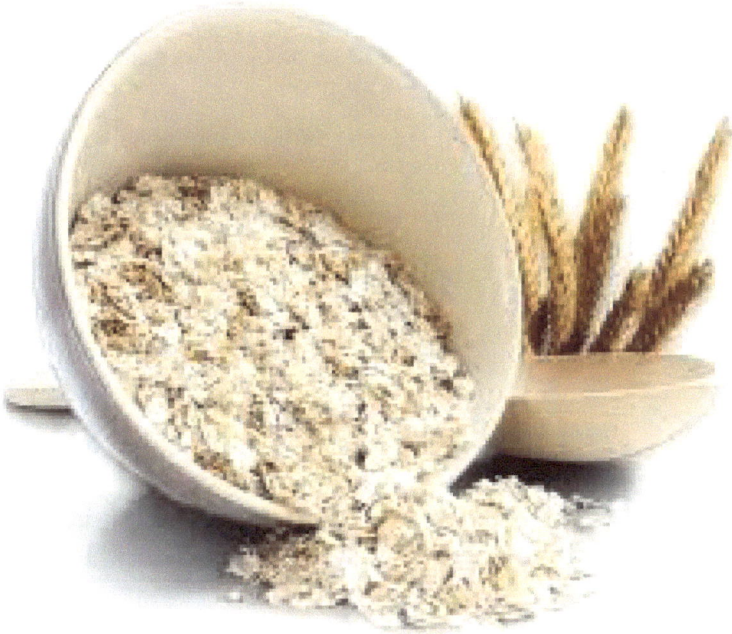

OATS are incredibly nutritious food packed with important vitamins, minerals and antioxidants. They are a good source of carbs and fiber. Oats are high in antioxidants called avenanthramides which aides in lowering the production of nitric oxide. In addition, avenanthramides have anti-inflammatory and anti-itching effects. They can lower cholesterol levels and protect LDL cholesterol from damage. Oats promote weight loss and aides in skin care. They also decrease the risk of childhood asthma. Oats may help relieve constipation.

WILD RICE

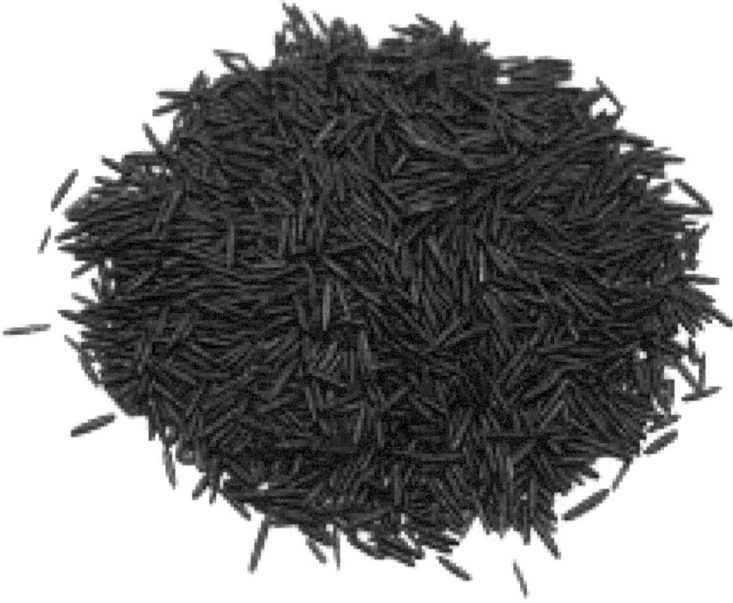

WILD RICE is both a protein and an anti-oxidant. It is much healthier than white rice. Eating wild rice will improve your mood and heart. Also, it is known for lowering the risk of Type 2 Diabetes. *"My family*

loves wild rice over sautéed vegetables."

"HERBS & ROOTS"

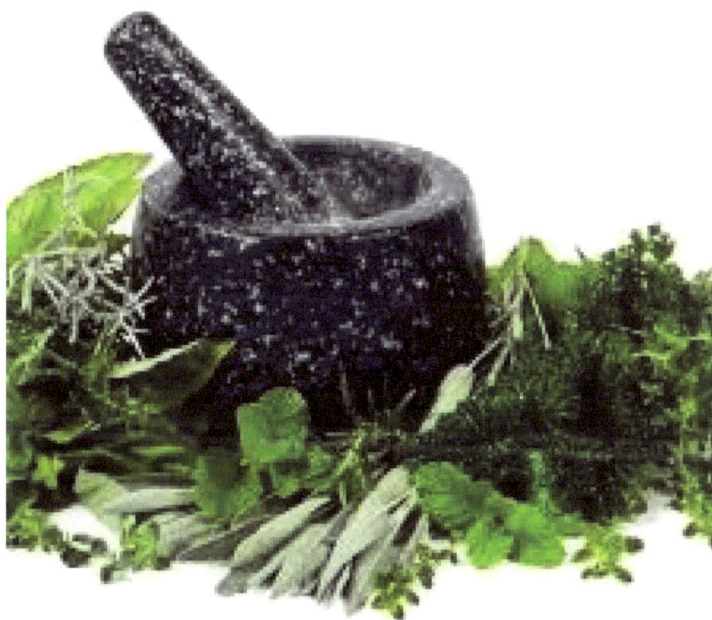

BASIL

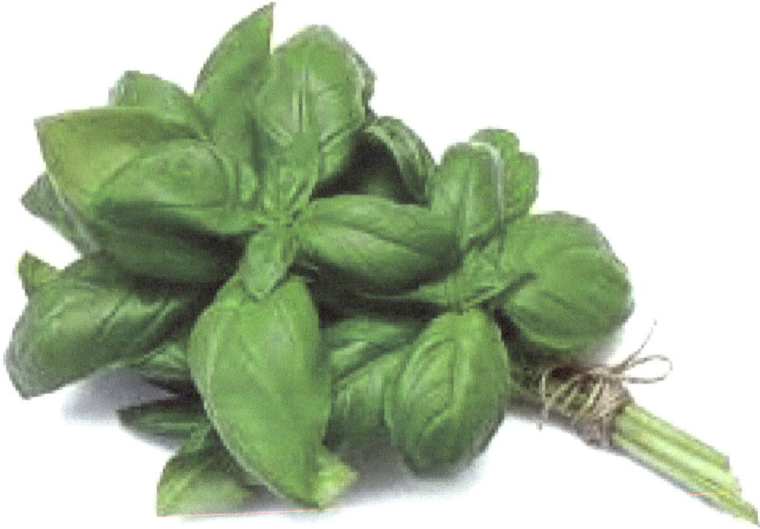

BASIL is a culinary herb of the mint family. It was found in mummies in Egypt because the ancient Egyptians used this herb for embalming. It has been known as an antidote for snake bites, colds, and inflammation within nasal passages. Basil may provide health benefits in the diet, as herbal medicine, and as an essential oil. It provides some macronutrients, such as calcium and vitamin K, as well as a range of antioxidants. Basil reduces oxidative stress. It supports liver health and helps fight cancer. Basil also protects against skin aging. It reduces high blood sugar and supports cardiovascular health. Basil boosts mental health, alleviating stress, anxiety, and depression. It increases the ability to think and prevents age-related memory loss. Basil also improves stress-related sleep and sex issues.

BEET ROOT

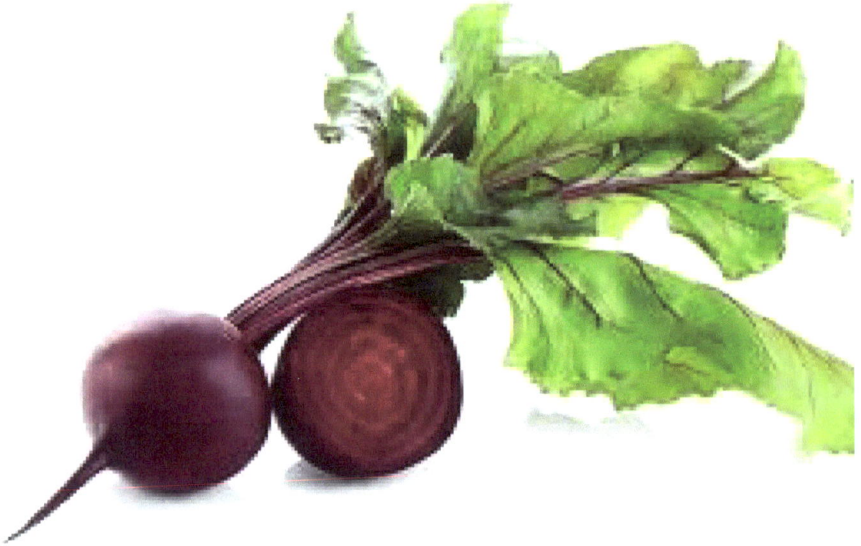

BEET ROOTS are packed with essential nutrients. They are a great source of fiber, folate, manganese, potassium, iron, and vitamin C. Beet roots have been associated with numerous health benefits including blood flow, lowering blood pressure, and increased exercise performance. It also aides in fighting inflammation. Boot roots improve digestive health, support brain heath and have some anti-cancer fighting properties. Because they are low in calories and high in water, they help to keep you hydrated. The fiber in beets may also help promote weight loss by reducing the appetite and promoting feelings of fullness, thereby reducing overall calorie intake.

GINGER

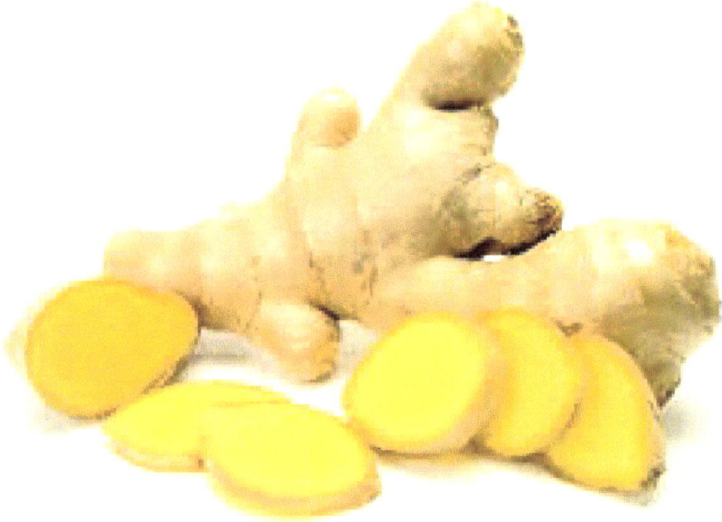

GINGER is actually a rhizome, not a root. The ginger plant is an herb. Ginger has many health benefits, some including anti-inflammatory properties, blood sugar regulation, and gastrointestinal relief. It reduces muscle pain and soreness. Ginger has been known to treat many forms of nausea, especially morning sickness. It also aides in chronic indigestion. Ginger significantly reduces menstrual pain. Ginger contains a substance that may help to prevent cancer. It improves brain function and protects against Alzheimer's disease.

PARSLEY

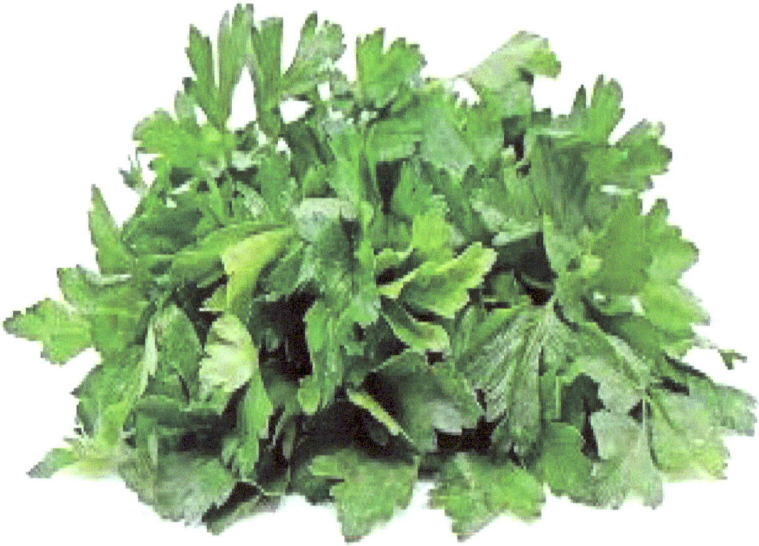

PARSLEY is a flowering plant native to the Mediterranean. The two most common types are French curly-leaf and Italian flat-leaf which is pictured above. This herb is rich in many vitamins, particularly vitamin K, which is needed for blood clotting and bone health. It also contains vitamins A and C.

Parsley is very low in calories, yet it packs a powerful punch with flavor. It is also rich in antioxidants. Parsley contains cancer-fighting substances. It is rich in nutrients that protect your eyes and improves heart health. You can incorporate dried or fresh leaves easily into your diet by adding it to soups, salads, marinades, and sauces.

TUMERIC

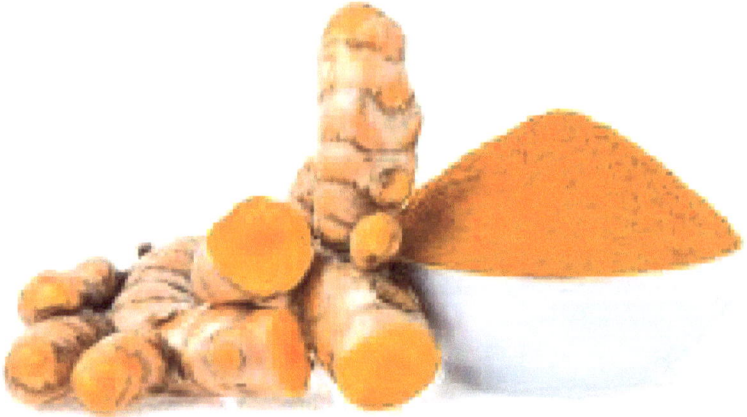

TUMERIC is a powerful superfood that is medicinal. It contains bioactive compounds with healing properties. Because it is an antioxidant with super powers, it can enhance the body quickly. Tumeric also serves as a natural pain reliever. It aides in digestion and gives our bodies liver support. It is a good source of vitamin C, magnesium, iron, and potassium. Tumeric can be used for moderate skin care, especially for pimples and is often used for reducing inflammation. It may help to reduce pain from arthritis. It will also assist in lowering your cholesterol. Tumeric can be use to boost cognitive abilities.

"OTHER"

ALEO VERA PLANT

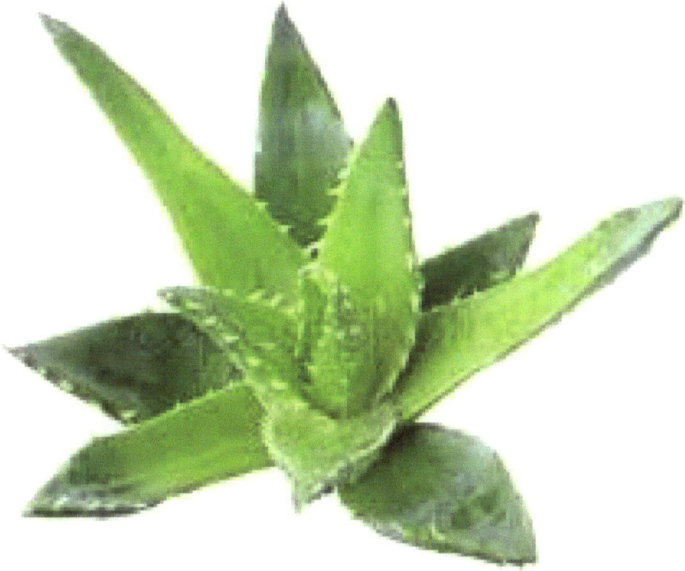

ALEO VERA PLANTS are a popular medicinal plant that has been used for thousands of years. Its leaves are full of a gel-like substance that contains numerous beneficial compounds. The aloe vera plants have various powerful antioxidants that can help inhibit the growth of harmful bacteria. It accelerates the healing of burns, reduces dental plaque, and helps treat canker sores. Aloe vera has often been used to treat constipation as well. It improves the skin and prevent wrinkles. It lowers blood sugar levels too!

CHIA SEEDS

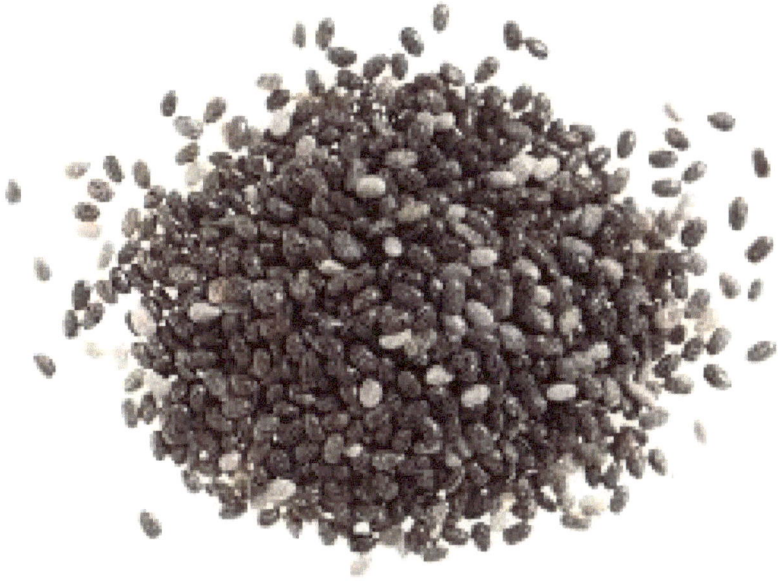

CHIA SEEDS deliver a massive amount of nutrients with very few calories. "Chia" is an ancient Mayan word for "strength." They are loaded with antioxidants that fight off the production of free radicals. Almost all the carbs in chia seeds are fiber. Chia seeds are high in quality protein. They are the most weight loss friendly dietary nutrient. Chia seeds are very high in omega-3 fatty acids. They lower your risk of heart disease and significantly reduce blood pressure in people with hypertension, which is a strong risk factor for heart disease. They are important for bone health too. Chia seeds reduces blood sugar levels and chronic inflammation.

CINNAMON STICK

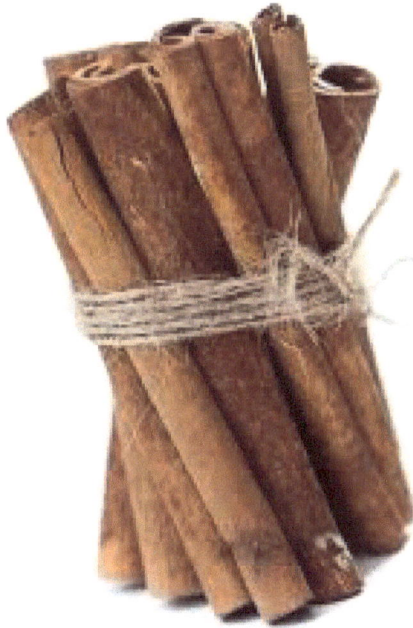

CINNAMON STICKS are the second most popular spice after black pepper. It is commonly used as a supplement to treat problems with the digestive system, diabetes, loss of appetite, and other conditions. It has also been used in traditional medicine for Bronchitis. Cinnamon may also help treat some types of fungal infections. Studies have suggested that cinnamon may help the prevention of Alzeheimer's disease and help to protect against the HIV infection. It also contain inflammatory properties as well.

FLAXSEEDS

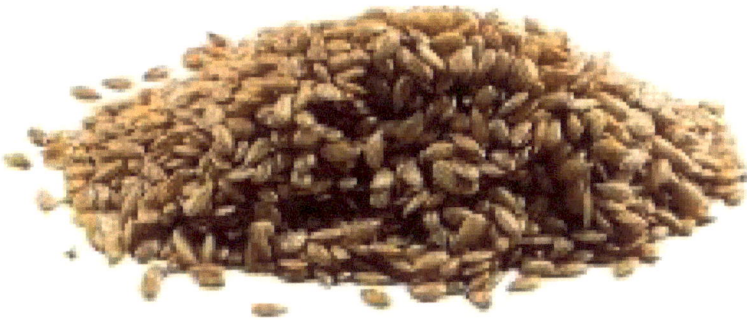

FLAXSEEDS have been praised for their health-protective properties. Just one tablespoon provides a good amount of protein, fiber, and omega-3 fatty acids, in addition to being a rich source of vitamins and minerals. Flaxseeds aide in reducing the risk of cancer. It improves your overall cholesterol levels and lowers your blood pressure. Flaxseeds contain a high-quality protein. They help control blood sugar. Flaxseeds keep hunger at bay, which may aide in weight control.

GREEN TEA

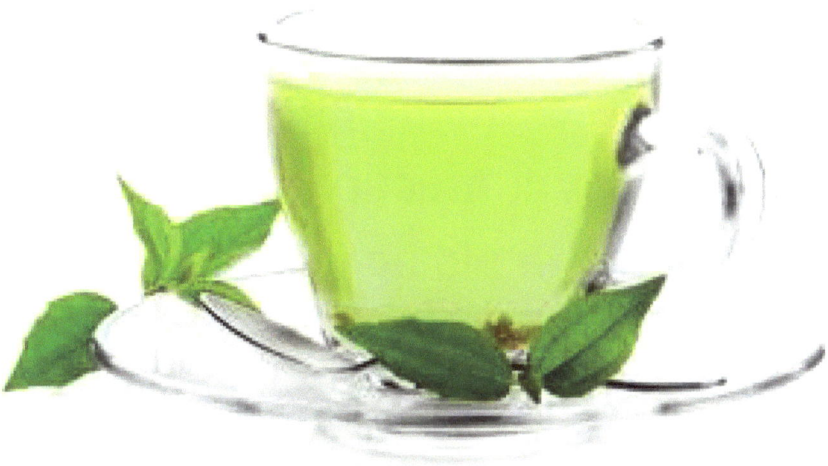

GREEN TEA is the healthiest beverage on the planet! It is loaded with antioxidants and nutrients that have powerful effects on the body. These include improved brain function, fat loss, a lower risk of cancer and many other impressive benefits. Green tea is rich in polyphenols that have effects like reducing inflammation and helping to fight cancer. It improves physical performance as well. Green tea aides in killing bacteria, which improves dental health and lowers your risk of infection. It protects your brain in old age, lowering your risk of Alzheimer's and Parkinson's diseases. It also lowers the risk of Type 2 Diabetes and reduces the risk of Cardiovascular disease. Green tea can help you lose weight and lower your risk of obesity. This powerful drink help you live longer!

HONEY

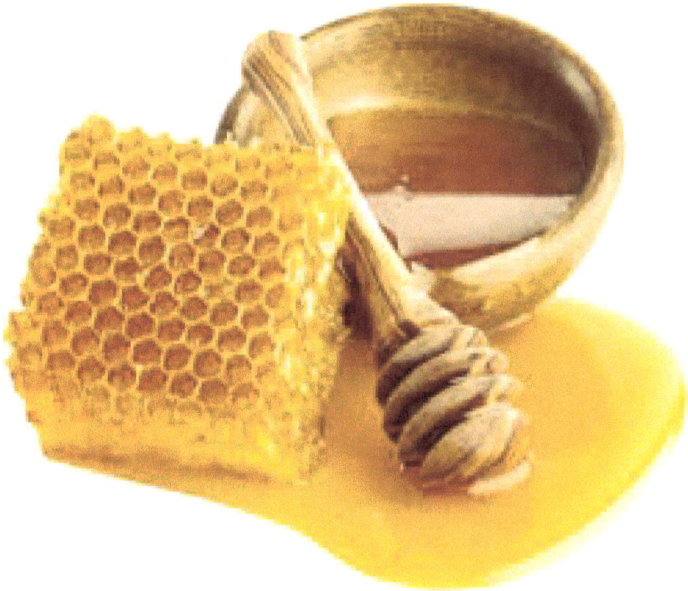

HONEY since ancient times have been used as both food and medicine. High quality honey is rich in antioxidants. The antioxidants in honey can help to lower your blood pressure which is an important risk factor for heart disease. Honey also improves cholesterol. It leads to modest reductions in total and "bad" LDL cholesterol while raising "good" HDL cholesterol. It promotes burn and wound healing. It also suppresses coughs in children. Honey is the sugar substitute for a Diabetic as studies show that honey can lower triglyceride levels.

MUSHROOM

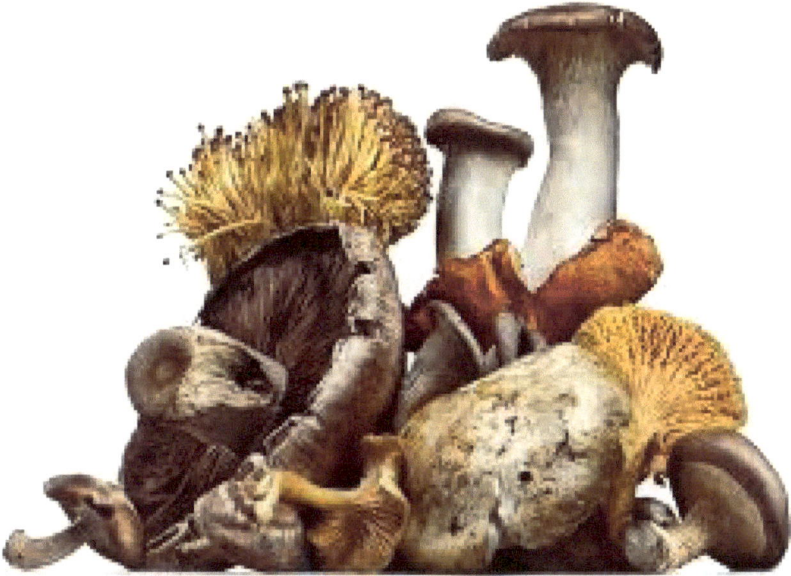

MUSHROOMS are high in antioxidants. They are known as an anti-aging food. Many believe the mushrooms are a vegetable, but it isn't. It is a *fungus*. I use mushrooms as a meat substitute as it is known as the "meat" of the vegetable world. A single mushroom can contain more potassium than a banana. It is loaded with vitamin B. Mushrooms are made up of around 90% water. They also contain medicinal properties.

In Corinthians: 6:19-20

Or do you know that your body is a temple of the holy spirit within you, whom you have from God? You are not your own, for you were bought with a price. So glorify God in you body.

In Genesis 1:29

And God said, "Behold, I have given you every plant yielding seeds that is on the face of all the earth, and every tree with seeds in its fruit. You shall have them for food.

The Four Elements

Earth, Air, Water, and Fire

Each Represent 90° Degrees

Which equals out to a square.

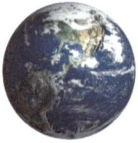

Earth 90°

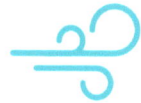

Air 90°

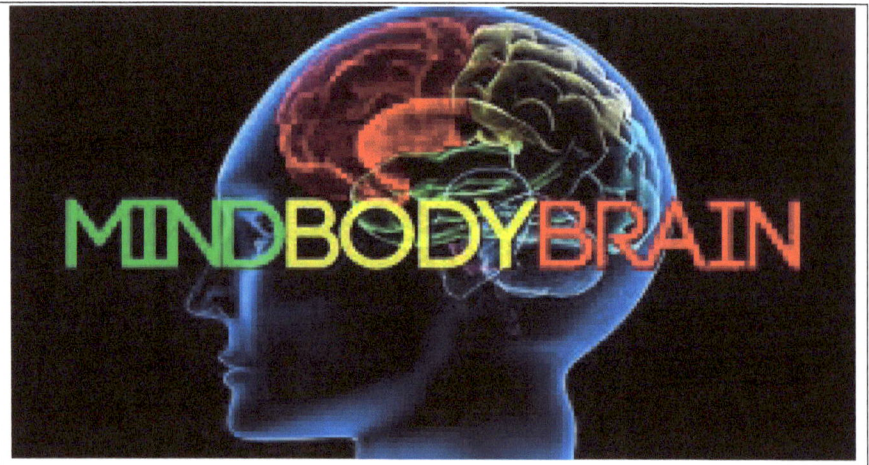

Water 90°

Fire 90°

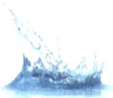

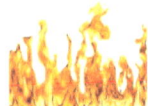

Plant food can never come into existence without an Earth to grow on Element 1. Earth is 1/4th land... an ancient intelligent element. "Earth" is 90° degrees in the square of the four elements.

In order for plant food to grow, it needs air in both the soil and environment which is Element 2. "Air" is an ancient intelligent element that sits on a 90° degree angle as well.

All plant food is totally reliant on "water" which is Element 3. This ancient intelligent elements lovers ¾ water. Water on the scale of on of the ancient intelligent element is also 90° degrees.

Fire or Sun is another intelligent ancient element plant food wouldn't thrive if no sun was alive. The "Sun" and "Fire" is 90° Degrees on the scale of the four elements.

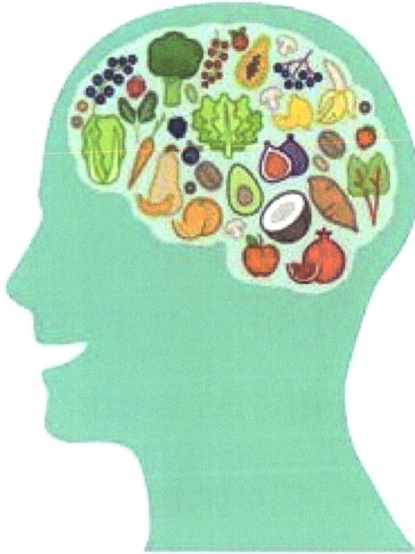

These intelligent ancient element properties go directly into the plant based foods.

When you eat foods from PLANTS and PLANT BASED. These foods are ELECTRIC which charge your ELECTRICAL BODY and mind now because these 4 elements are both ancient and intelligent when you eat them, you are eating ancient intelligent elements and if you are exclusively eating them or predominately eating plant based. Those intelligent elements will advance your spiritual MIND and optimize your ultimate driving machine which is the body.

Man lived to be 200, 300, 400, 500, 600 years old/ but when many got away from a plant-based diet became the prime source of people food. People started dying at 40, 50, 60, 70, 80, and 90 years old with body parts removed, pills and side affects and ills galore. People are dying prematurely!

Now back to the four elements:

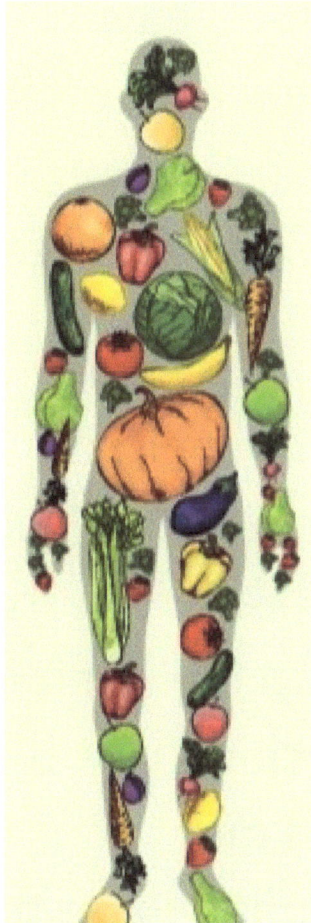

.....Super natural people pose the greatest threat to the sickness that's being sold to people, so it's important that they inform you with unhealthy food eating...So they say! As a result, animal eating is advertised so heavily! Because if you are eating a lot of dead cooked animals, sickness is sure to start the following with disease...

Diseases sell period! It keeps a particular group of people very wealthy while misinforming most on how to fuel their ultimate driving machine (the body), so let superfoods meet your taste buds and let your lips share the words of love health, wealth, and "know thyself" with others and stay fresh off the vine!

Plant food is electric and so are you!

Eating healthy is done one bite at a time!

Rise more in love with yourself and add more superfoods to your diet to ensure longevity in your lifetime. Love your animals, not eat them!

Superfoods alter your mood, they make you calm, and enhance your body and mind. They are loaded with mega power proteins, antioxidants, nutrients, minerals, and more. You can find these superfoods in your local grocery store.

God is activated inside of you. Let this year be the year that you grow into wellness. I hope that you enjoyed walking your mind and eyes across this "Holy Book of Superfoods."

THE END

ABOUT THE AUTHOR

Antonio Ford, "The Food Lord" has published 5 books and 1 DVD to date. Antonio has taken a personal interest in helping others fight the battle of eating healthy "One-Day-At-A-Time". He has committed his life to providing information to all humans.

www.ingramcontent.com/pod-product-compliance
Lightning Source LLC
Chambersburg PA
CBHW040131270326
41929CB00001B/3